Eosinophilic Esophagitis

Cookbook For Seniors Over 50

Gastronomic Delights: Culinary Treasures for Senior Digestion

Rhonda C Anderson MS RDN

Contents

Conclusion.

Introduction

Introducing Mabel, a lively 78-year-old grandma who has been bravely facing the difficulties posed by Eosinophilic Esophagitis (EoE), a chronic immune system illness that has been inflaming her esophagus. Mabel has been dealing with her illness for a long time, and it has caused her emotional and psychological anguish in addition to physical pain.

Mabel struggled silently, suffering from excruciating chest pain and difficulties swallowing, while living alone. Her secret was never shared until her son-in-law and devoted daughter made her an unannounced visit. They consulted a reliable family friend for guidance since they were worried and wanted to help, and the friend suggested getting professional aid.

At that point, I intervened, equipped with a plethora of information and a customized strategy derived from the "Eosinophilic Esophagitis Cookbook for Seniors." Understanding that older people, such as Mabel, have certain nutritional requirements, I developed a detailed plan to help her feel better and regain her energy.

Mabel set out on a transforming path toward recovery with her family. With commitment and persistence, they adopted wholesome foods and professional advice, and they saw incredible results as Mabel started to restore her vitality and strength.

Through poignant discussions and personal anecdotes, Mabel's family solidified their position as champions of the role that a healthy diet plays in preventing EoE in older adults. Their testimonials are a source of inspiration for anyone facing comparable difficulties in their senior years.

You are not alone in this trip, seniors and their families facing the harsh reality of the End of the

Earth. Purchasing resources such as the "Eosinophilic Esophagitis Cookbook for Seniors" is an essential first step in recovering one's health and physical state.

Turning the pages of this priceless guide will reveal not only mouthwatering recipes but also empowering thoughts and useful advice to help you create a more vibrant, happier future. Let us work together to find the solution that will enable elderly people like Mabel to age gracefully and vibrantly and to live happy, fulfilling lives.

Chapter 1

Understanding Eosinophilic Esophagitis

What is Eosinophilic Esophagitis?

An allergic reaction that affects the esophagus is called eosinophilic esophagitis. The esophagus becomes irritated and has improper contractions. It may get constricted and form abscesses or rings. Your immune system produces white blood cells in response to an allergen, which causes the symptoms. The term "eosinophil" refers to the white blood cells.

The illness is referred to as eosinophilic esophagitis, or EoE for short. It commonly affects white males and can occur at any age.

Symptoms and Diagnosis

Each person experiences EoE symptoms differently, however they can include:

- Trouble swallowing
- Chest pain or heartburn
- Abdominal pain
- Vomiting
- Food getting stuck in the throat due to narrowing (this is a medical emergency)
- Stunted growth or poor weight gain in children

Diagnosis

In addition to taking your medical history, your healthcare professional probably wants to do an allergy test. An endoscopy by a gastroenterologist, a specialist in digestive (stomach and swallowing) diseases, is likely to be requested by him or her. A tiny, flexible endoscope with a camera is passed into your mouth and down your throat during this outpatient treatment to examine your esophagus. The gastroenterologist will look for elevated eosinophil counts and outward manifestations of inflammation. Your gastroenterologist will probably need to take a biopsy, or tissue sample, from your esophagus in order to confirm the diagnosis.

Treatment

You will have to collaborate closely with a gastroenterologist or allergist to receive treatment. They will assist you in identifying substances or foods to stay away from. While there isn't a single medication that may treat EoE, several medications, such corticosteroids and proton pump inhibitors, as well as avoiding some foods, like dairy, eggs, wheat, soy, peanuts, tree nuts, and fish, can help lessen esophageal redness and swelling.

Finding out what triggers your allergic reaction and avoiding it will help you manage EoE. Allergens are frequently derived from food. It's also critical to understand that reactions to EoE may not manifest for days or weeks at a time. Remember this when you start a food elimination program. If you are avoiding a certain food, it may take some time to see if it was a successful tactic.

If the esophagus has narrowed, it may occasionally need to be dilated, or stretched.

Complications

We don't fully understand the long-term effects of EoE. If treatment is not received, the symptoms may worsen and the esophagus may become damaged and narrowed.

Living With EoE

It's critical to collaborate closely with your gastroenterologist to manage EoE. When testing is necessary to determine if your EoE is improving or declining, he or she can advise you on this. Dietitians and allergists/immunologists can assist you in managing linked issues such as food allergies, allergic rhinitis, and asthma. Collaborate with your medical providers so that they can communicate with one another. Support groups and organizations might be beneficial for certain families. An group called the American Partnership for Eosinophilic Disorders (APFED) assists families in managing EoE.

Impact on Seniors Over 50

1. Age-Related Complications: Seniors over 50 may already be coping with a number of medical issues, such as diabetes, arthritis, or hypertension. Their health management becomes much more challenging as a result of EoE.

Because some EoE treatments may interfere with routinely prescribed medications for seniors, the presence of EoE can worsen pre-existing diseases or make medication management more difficult.

2. Nutritional Challenges: Elderly people with end-of-life encounter dysphagia, which can result in inadequate food consumption and malnourishment. Their general health and quality of life may be further impacted by this.

The stringent nature of elimination of common allergens (EoE) diets can be especially difficult for seniors who may already be on restricted diets because of other health issues.

3.Psychological Impact: Seniors' mental health may suffer as a result of managing the dietary limitations and symptoms of end-of-life anxiety, which may result in emotions of despair, annoyance, or loneliness.

Anxiety regarding the possible side effects of end-of-life issues, like esophageal strictures or the requirement for invasive operations like esophageal dilatation, is another common concern among seniors.

4.   Healthcare   Access   and Communication: Seniors may experience difficulties getting to healthcare facilities due to decreased mobility, transportation problems, or budgetary limitations. These obstacles may make it more difficult for them to get an early diagnosis and treatment for EoE.

Managing EoE requires seniors and their healthcare providers to have effective communication. Clear and patient-centered communication tactics are necessary since elders may have difficulty expressing their symptoms or comprehending medical language.

5. Social Implications: Seniors with end-of-life experience may find it difficult to engage in food-related social activities, such as dinner parties with friends or family. Feelings of social alienation and isolation may result from this.

Family members and caregivers can foster a supportive environment and reduce stigma and misunderstanding by receiving education about EoE and its effects on seniors.

6. Treatment Considerations: When choosing a course of action for EoE in seniors, it's important to consider possible drug interactions as well as age-related health issues.

Although proton pump inhibitors (PPIs) and dietary changes are frequently employed to treat EoE, seniors may need individualized treatment regimens catered to their particular medical requirements and preferences.

Chapter 2

The Senior's Guide to Eating with EoE

Diet Restrictions and Triggers

1. Elimination Diet: Removing particular foods that are known to cause allergic reactions is part of an elimination diet, which is one of the main strategies for treating EoE. Symptoms of EoE can be made worse by common allergens such as dairy, wheat, soy, eggs, nuts, and seafood. Seniors who want to build an elimination plan specific to their requirements and preferences should collaborate with a nutritionist or healthcare specialist.

2. Soft Foods: EoE-affected seniors may experience comfort by eating softer, more easily ingested foods. Tender meats, well-cooked grains, and pureed fruits and vegetables can all be easy on the esophagus and less irritating. Steer clear of coarse or scratchy materials to assist stop the inflammation from getting worse.

3. Acidic and Spicy Foods: By irritating the esophagus, acidic foods like citrus fruits, tomatoes, and vinegar, as well as spicy meals, can worsen the symptoms of oedema. In order to lessen discomfort and inflammation, seniors should restrict or stay away from these kinds of foods.

4. Food Additives: People with EoE may experience adverse responses in response to specific food additives and preservatives. Ingredients like artificial flavors, colors, and preservatives that are frequently found in processed foods should be avoided by seniors.

Choosing unprocessed, less processed foods might lessen the possibility of setting off symptoms.

5. Dietary Fiber: Although fiber is necessary for a healthy digestive system, some elderly people with EoE may discover that meals heavy in fiber, such as whole grains and legumes, exacerbate their symptoms. In these situations, it may be advantageous to select low-fiber substitutes such white rice or refined grains.

6. Allergen Testing: To pinpoint particular triggers that exacerbate their symptoms, seniors with EoE may find relief through allergy testing. They can more successfully adjust their diet to avoid troublesome foods and manage their condition by identifying allergens.

Triggers:

1. Environmental Allergens: For those who are vulnerable, pollen, dust mites, pet dander, and other environmental allergens can worsen the symptoms of oedema. Seniors can reduce their exposure to these triggers by utilizing air purifiers, maintaining a clean living environment, and limiting their interaction with recognized allergens.

2. Stress and worry: By impacting the immune system and digestive systems, emotional stress and worry can either cause or exacerbate symptoms in the early stages of EOE. Seniors can assist manage their health holistically by engaging in stress-reduction practices like deep breathing, meditation, and light exercise.

3. Texture and Temperature: Extreme heat or cold can aggravate the esophagus and cause symptoms in elderly people who have eoE. Similarly, abrasive or rough food textures can also lead to pain and inflammation. Avoiding exacerbating the illness can be achieved by selecting softer textures and eating meals at reasonable temperatures.

4. Medication Interactions: Certain pharmaceuticals, especially antibiotics and nonsteroidal anti-inflammatory drugs (NSAIDs), have the potential to exacerbate the symptoms of encephalitis or to conflict with the course of treatment. Seniors should speak with their doctor to make sure that their prescriptions aren't aggravating their illness, and if necessary, they should look into other options.

Tips for Meal Planning and Preparation

1. Plan Like a Pro: Incorporate weekly exploration into your meal preparation. It's similar to setting out on a less stressful, healthier gastronomic adventure!

2. Create Your Culinary Canvas: See your entire week as a masterful menu. Draw up your meals using a vibrant palette of tastes and nutrients from sunrise to sunset.

3. Balance Is Key: Visualize your meal as a well-balanced mixture of healthy fats, proteins, and carbohydrates. For a masterpiece of nutrition, combine a rainbow of fruits, vegetables, whole grains, lean meats, and healthy fats.

4. List it, Love it: Convert your grocery list into a dinner plan. It's your pass to a refrigerator and pantry full of food, protecting you from the lure of impulsive purchases.

5. Prepare Ahead, Unwind Later: Prepare meats, chop vegetables, and prepare grains ahead of time. It's like preparing your kitchen for the hectic week ahead by filling it with time-saving treasures.

6. Batch Up Brilliance: Prepare large quantities of delicious food that you can share and conquer. Store them in the fridge or freezer for convenient access to delicious handmade food during busy days.

7. Container Couture: Use high-quality containers to up your storage game. Glass ones keep your ready ingredients and leftovers safe and sound, just like the VIP section.

8. Time-Saving Magic: Unleash the potential of appliances that save time. Air fryers, quick pots, and slow cookers are culinary wizards that can create great food with very little work.

9. Simplicity Pleases: Don't be too complicated, foolish! Not every dinner has to be a work of art. Put an emphasis on simple dishes that are flavorful without being complicated.

10. Flavor Adventures: Take a risk and experiment with various cuisines and flavors. Try new recipes or give your old favorites a flavor boost with a pinch of herbs and spices.

11. Accept Flexibility: You have to wing it sometimes in life, just like in a recipe. Make adjustments to your meal plan as needed and roll with the punches. Being flexible is essential in life!

12. Savor the Experience: Cooking is a feast for the senses as well as a means of nourishing your body. Savor the pleasure of preparing tasty, wholesome meals that satisfy the body and the spirit. Savor each bite, sizzle, and chop!

Overcoming Challenges in Dining Out

Eosinophilic esophagitis (EoE) can make eating out difficult, particularly for elderly people. This is a thorough advice on how to get beyond these obstacles and still enjoy eating out:

1. Communication is Key: It's crucial to communicate with restaurant employees when dining out. It should be acceptable for seniors with EoE to inquire about menu items, preparation techniques, and possible cross-contamination hazards. Meals should be safe and appropriate for their nutritional needs, and this may be ensured with clear communication.

2. Planning and Research: Seniors can look up menus online or give a call in advance to find out which restaurants are EoE-friendly. Seek out eateries that can customize their menu items or that are open to meeting unique dietary needs.

3.Advocate for Accommodations:
When dining out, seniors should not be afraid to stand up for themselves. If a restaurant is unable to meet their dietary requirements, they may kindly ask for an alternative menu item or make a modification request.

4.Seniors who suffer from inflammatory bowel disease (EoE) should be mindful of typical trigger foods and components that can aggravate their symptoms. They can make educated decisions when dining out by staying away from recognized triggers like dairy, gluten, soy, and specific spices.

5.Portion Control: When dining out, elders should exercise portion control because overindulging can exacerbate signs of early aging. Reducing the amount of food you eat or eating with others can help avoid pain and digestive problems.

6.Bring Safe Snacks: When dining out, seniors can bring safe snacks in case their options are restricted or there are unforeseen delays. This guarantees that they will always have an alternative in the event that there are no acceptable meal selections.

7. Select Safe Cuisine: Some cuisines might be more tolerant of the EoE's dietary requirements than others. Seniors can look into vegetarian, Japanese, or Mediterranean food, which frequently uses simpler, more allergy-friendly ingredients.

8.Remain Hydrated: Elderly people with EoE should drink enough water to aid with symptoms like dry mouth and difficulty swallowing. To facilitate comfort and aid in digestion, encourage water consumption before, during, and following meals.

9. Mindful Eating Practices: To reduce symptoms and avoid overindulging, seniors should engage in mindful eating practices. To ensure optimal digestion, chew food slowly and thoroughly, take tiny chunks, and wait between bites.

Chapter 3

Delicious Breakfasts to Start Your Day Right

1.Banana Oat Cookies.

Prep Time:10 mins
Cook Time:15 mins
Total Time: 25 mins
Servings:12

Ingredients
- 2 bananas, mashed
- ¼ cup milk
- 1 large egg, beaten
- 1 teaspoon honey
- ½ teaspoon vanilla extract
- 1 cup rolled oats, or as needed

- 1 teaspoon ground cinnamon
- ½ teaspoon baking powder
- ⅛ teaspoon salt

Directions

1. Set the oven's temperature to 350°F, or 175°C. Use parchment paper to line a baking sheet.

2. In a bowl, combine mashed bananas, milk, egg, honey, and vanilla. Add the baking powder, cinnamon, oats, and salt and stir until thoroughly mixed. If the batter is too runny, add extra oats.

3. Spoon batter into mounds on the prepared baking sheet, spacing them a few inches apart.

4. Bake for about 15 minutes, or until the sides are golden and the tops appear dry.

Nutritional value

Calories=55
Fat=1g
Carbs=10g

Protein =2g

2. Banana Zucchini Bread

Prep Time:15 mins
Cook Time:45 mins
Total Time: 1hr
Servings:20

Ingredients
- 3 large eggs
- 1 cup white sugar
- 1 cup grated zucchini
- ¾ cup vegetable oil
- 2 bananas, mashed
- ⅔ cup packed brown sugar
- 2 teaspoons vanilla extract
- 3 ½ cups all-purpose flour
- 1 tablespoon ground cinnamon
- 1 ½ teaspoons baking powder
- 1 teaspoon baking soda

- 1 teaspoon salt
- ½ cup dried cranberries
- ½ cup chopped walnuts

Directions

1. Set the oven's temperature to 325°F, or 165°C. Line two 8x4-inch bread loaf pans with grease and flour.

2. Using an electric mixer, beat eggs in a large bowl until they are light yellow and foamy. Beat together white sugar, oil, zucchini, bananas, brown sugar, and vanilla. Add the salt, baking powder, baking soda, cinnamon, and flour and stir. Stir in the nuts and cranberries. Evenly divide the batter among the loaf pans that have been prepped.

3. Bake for 45 to 50 minutes, or until a toothpick inserted in the center comes out clean, in the preheated oven. Before taking them out and serving, let them cool in the loaf pans on a wire rack.

Nutritional value

Calories=272
Fat=10g
Carbs=40g
Protein =4g

3.Rhonda Special Scrambled

Prep Time:15 mins
Cook Time:20 mins
Total Time: 35 mins
Servings:6

Ingredients
- 2 tablespoons olive oil
- 2 pounds ground beef
- 2 medium onions, chopped
- 1 (8 ounce) package sliced fresh mushrooms
- 2 cloves garlic, minced

- 1 (10 ounce) package frozen chopped spinach, thawed and drained
- ½ teaspoon ground nutmeg
- ½ teaspoon dried oregano
- salt and pepper to taste
- 6 large eggs, beaten

Directions

1. In a large skillet, heat the oil over medium-high heat. Add the ground beef and cook, stirring, for about 8 minutes, or until browned and crumbly. After draining any surplus oil, mix in the garlic, onions, and mushrooms. For approximately five minutes, or until the onion has softened and become translucent, reduce the heat to medium, cover, and cook. Add the spinach, nutmeg, oregano, salt, and pepper. Cook for 3 to 4 minutes, or until the spinach is well heated.

2. Set the temperature on medium-low. Add the eggs to the skillet and cook, scrambling, for 4 to 6 minutes, or until cooked to your preference

and combined with the beef and spinach combination.

Tips

Instead of making scrambled eggs, use the back of a spoon to create six wells in the beef and spinach mixture after lowering the heat in Step 2. Place one egg into each well, cover, and cook for four to six minutes, or until the eggs are done to your preference.

4.Avocado Spinach Dip

Prep Time:15 mins
Additional Time: 1hr
Total Time: 1 hr 15mins
Servings:8

Ingredients

- 2 cups fresh spinach
- 1 cup diced avocado
- ½ cup reduced-fat sour cream
- ¼ cup chopped red onion
- 1 tablespoon chopped seeded jalapeno pepper
- ½ teaspoon salt
- ⅛ teaspoon ground black pepper
- hot sauce

Directions

1. In a food processor, blend together spinach, avocado, sour cream, red onion, jalapeño pepper, salt, black pepper, and spicy sauce until smooth.

2. Scrape the dip into a serving bowl, place plastic wrap over it, and chill it for at least an hour.

Nutritional value

Calories=56
Fat=5g
Carbs=3g
Protein =1g

5.Quinoa porridge

Prep Time:5 mins
Cook Time: 30 mins
Total Time: 35 mins
Servings:3

Ingredients

- ½ cup quinoa
- ¼ teaspoon ground cinnamon
- 1 ½ cups almond milk
- ½ cup water
- 2 tablespoons brown sugar
- 1 teaspoon vanilla extract (Optional)
- 1 pinch salt

Directions

1. Add the quinoa to a pot that has been heated to medium heat. Add cinnamon for seasoning and cook, stirring often, until toasted, about 3 minutes. After adding the water, vanilla, and almond milk, whisk in the salt and brown sugar. After bringing to a boil, reduce the heat and simmer for about 25 minutes, or until the porridge is thick and the grains are soft. If the liquid has dried up before the food is done cooking, add more water as needed. Stir from time to time, especially toward the end, to avoid scorching.

Nutritional value

Calories=173
Fat=3g
Carbs=31g
Protein =4g

6.Asparagus with Sliced Almonds and Parmesan Cheese

Prep Time:2 mins
Cook Time: 10 mins
Total Time: 12 mins
Servings:3

Ingredients
- 2 tablespoons butter
- 1 pound asparagus, bottoms trimmed
- ⅓ cup sliced almonds
- ⅓ cup Parmesan cheese

Directions
1. In a large skillet over medium-high heat, melt butter. Add the asparagus and simmer for about 3 minutes while stirring. Add the almonds and parmesan, then simmer for 3 to 5 minutes, or until the cheese starts to color slightly.

Nutritional value

Calories=178

Fat=14g

Carbs=7g

Protein =8g

7.Buckwheat pancakes

Prep Time:10 mins

Cook Time: 10 mins

Additional Time: 5 mins

Total Time: 25 mins

Servings:4

Ingredients

- 1 cup buckwheat flour
- 1 ½ teaspoons white sugar
- 1 teaspoon baking powder
- ¼ teaspoon baking soda
- ¼ teaspoon salt

- 1 ¼ cups buttermilk
- 1 large egg, beaten
- ¼ teaspoon vanilla extract
- 1 tablespoon unsalted butter, or as needed

Directions

1. In a larger bowl, whisk together buckwheat flour, sugar, baking powder, baking soda, and salt.

2. In a big basin, beat buttermilk, egg, and vanilla together.

3. Add flour mixture to buttermilk mixture and stir until smooth and thick batter is achieved. Give the batter time to settle and produce bubbles, approximately five minutes.

4. On a griddle set over medium heat, melt butter. Spoon the batter onto the heated griddle in large spoonfuls, and cook for 3 to 4 minutes, or until bubbles form and the edges dry. In 2 to 3 minutes, flip and continue cooking until the other side is browned. Proceed with the leftover batter.

5. Accompany with berries.

Nutritional value

Calories=196
Fat=6g
Carbs=26g
Protein =9g

8.Chia seed pudding

Prep Time:15 mins
Additional Time: 8 hrs 30 mins
Total Time: 8 hrs 45 mins
Servings:4

Ingredients
- 1 cup unsweetened vanilla-flavored almond milk
- 1 cup vanilla fat-free yogurt

- 2 tablespoons pure maple syrup
- 1 teaspoon pure vanilla extract
- ⅛ teaspoon salt
- ¼ cup chia seeds
- 1 pint strawberries, hulled and chopped
- 4 teaspoons pure maple syrup
- ¼ cup toasted almonds

Directions

1. In a bowl, combine the almond milk, yogurt, two tablespoons maple syrup, vanilla, and salt. Whisk to mix well. Add the chia seeds and let soak for half an hour.

2. To disperse the seeds that have collected throughout the mixture, stir the chia seed mixture. Place plastic wrap over the bowl and chill for eight hours or overnight.

3. Place 4 teaspoons of maple syrup in a bowl with the strawberries and toss to coat. Stir the strawberries with the almonds.

4. Divide the chia seed mixture into four bowls and place some of the strawberry mixture on top of each.

Nutritional value

Calories=243
Fat=8g
Carbs=38g
Protein =7g

9.Gluten Free Buttermilk Pancakes

Prep Time:15 mins
Cook Time:20 mins
Total Time: 35 mins
Servings:10

Ingredients
- ½ cup brown rice flour

- ½ cup gluten-free all-purpose flour
- 3 tablespoons buckwheat flour
- 2 tablespoons white sugar
- 1 ¼ teaspoons baking powder
- 1 pinch baking soda
- 1 cup buttermilk, divided
- 2 medium eggs, separated
- 2 tablespoons light oil

Directions

1. In a bowl, whisk together sugar, baking powder, baking soda, brown rice flour, all-purpose flour, and buckwheat flour. In a separate basin, combine 3/4 cup buttermilk, egg yolks, and oil; stir until blended. To the buttermilk mixture, add the dry ingredients and whisk just until incorporated. Don't whisk the batter too much.

2. In a glass, metal, or ceramic bowl, beat the egg whites until soft peaks form. Whisk the egg whites into the mixture. The consistency of the

batter should be like tomato soup. If the batter is too thick, gradually add more buttermilk while giving it some time to set. (Gluten-free flours take a little longer to thicken; they take 45 to 1 minute to absorb the liquid.)

3. Turn up the heat to medium on a lightly greased griddle. Pour the batter onto the griddle in 1/4-cup portions. Simmer for 3 to 4 minutes, or until bubbles appear and the tops are beginning to get dry. In 2 to 3 minutes, flip and continue cooking until the other side is browned. Continue using the leftover batter.

4. Serve hot or hold off on freezing until fully chilled.

Nutritional value

Calories=114
Fat=4g
Carbs=16g
Protein =4g

10.Cottage Cheese Salad

Prep Time:10 mins
Total Time: 10 mins
Servings:4

Ingredients
- 1 (16 ounce) container cottage cheese, drained
- 4 roma (plum) tomatoes, chopped
- 4 green onions, chopped
- 2 medium cucumbers, peeled and diced
- salt and pepper, to taste

Directions
1. Combine the cottage cheese, tomatoes, cucumbers, and green onions in a medium-sized bowl. To taste, add salt and pepper for seasoning. Before serving, refrigerate.

Nutritional value

Calories=138
Fat=5g
Carbs=8g
Protein =15g

Chapter 4

Satisfying Soups, Salads, and Sides

1.Butternut squash soup

Prep Time:20 mins
Cook Time:45 mins
Total Time: 1 hrs 5 mins
Servings:4

Ingredients
- 2 tablespoons butter
- 1 small onion, chopped
- 1 stalk celery, chopped
- 1 medium carrot, chopped
- 2 medium potatoes, cubed

- 1 medium butternut squash - peeled, seeded, and cubed
- 1 (32 fluid ounce) container chicken stock
- salt and freshly ground black pepper to taste

Directions

1. Compile all of the ingredients.

2. In a large pot over medium heat, melt butter and sauté the onion, celery, carrot, potatoes, and squash for about 5 minutes, or until they are gently browned. Add enough chicken stock so that the vegetables are covered.

3. Place on medium-high heat and bring to a boil. After about 40 minutes, or until all the vegetables are soft, reduce the heat to low, cover the pot, and simmer.

4. Move the soup into a blender and blend until it's smooth. To get the appropriate consistency, return to the pot and stir in any leftover stock. Add pepper and salt for seasoning.

5. Present and savor

Nutritional value

Calories=305
Fat=7g
Carbs=60g
Protein =7g

2.Thai Coconut Soup

Prep Time:30 mins
Cook Time: 30 mins
Total Time: 1 hr
Servings:8

Ingredients

- 1 tablespoon vegetable oil
- 2 tablespoons grated fresh ginger
- 2 teaspoons red curry paste
- 1 stalk lemongrass, minced
- 4 cups chicken broth
- 3 tablespoons fish sauce
- 1 tablespoon light brown sugar
- 3 (13.5 ounce) cans coconut milk
- ½ pound fresh shiitake mushrooms, sliced
- 1 pound medium shrimp - peeled and deveined
- 2 tablespoons fresh lime juice
- salt to taste
- ¼ cup chopped fresh cilantro

Directions

1. Compile the ingredients.

2. Place a big pot over medium heat with oil. Stir in the lemongrass, ginger, and curry paste. Cook for one minute while stirring in the heated oil.

3.Slowly whisk in the chicken stock, followed by the brown sugar and fish sauce. Lower the heat and simmer for fifteen minutes.

4. Add the coconut milk and mushrooms. Cook, stirring, for about 5 minutes, or until the mushrooms are tender.

5.Cook the shrimp for about 5 minutes, or until they are no longer translucent. Add the lime juice, sprinkle with salt, and add the cilantro for garnish.

6. Have fun!

Nutritional value

Calories=368
Fat=33g
Carbs=9g
Protein =13g

3.Coconut Curry Pumpkin Soup

Prep Time: 20 mins
Additional Time: 30 mins
Total Time: 50 mins
Servings: 6

Ingredients

- ¼ cup coconut oil
- 1 cup chopped onions
- 3 cups vegetable broth
- 1 teaspoon curry powder
- ½ teaspoon salt
- ¼ teaspoon ground coriander
- ¼ teaspoon crushed red pepper flakes
- 1 (15 ounce) can 100% pure pumpkin
- 1 cup light coconut milk

Directions

1. In a big pot set over medium-high heat, warm the coconut oil. Add the onions and stir. Cook for about 5 minutes, or until the onions are transparent. Stir in the red pepper flakes, curry

powder, salt, and coriander. For around ten minutes, cook and stir the mixture until it gently boils. Continue boiling for another 15 to 20 minutes while stirring now and again. After whisking in the coconut milk and pumpkin, simmer for a further five minutes.

2. Transfer the soup to a blender, filling it only halfway, and mix in batches if needed, until the consistency is smooth. Before serving, transfer back to a pot and quickly reheat over medium heat.

Nutritional value

Calories=171
Fat=14g
Carbs=12g
Protein =2g

4.Quick and Vegetable Soup

Prep Time:15 mins
Cook Time: 35 mins
Total Time: 50 mins
Servings:6

Ingredients

- 1 (14.5 ounce) can diced tomatoes
- 1 (14 ounce) can chicken broth
- 1 (11.5 ounce) can tomato-vegetable juice cocktail
- 2 carrots, sliced
- 2 stalks celery, diced
- 1 large potato, diced
- 1 cup chopped fresh green beans
- 1 cup fresh corn kernels
- 1 cup water
- salt and pepper to taste
- 1 pinch Creole seasoning, or more to taste

Directions

1. Compile the ingredients.
2. In a large stockpot, combine tomatoes, celery, carrots, potatoes, green beans, corn, and water. Also add chicken broth and tomato juice. Add salt, pepper, and Creole seasoning for flavor.
3. Bring to a boil over medium heat, then simmer for about 30 minutes, or until vegetables are cooked.
4. Present warm and savor.

Nutritional value

Calories=116
Fat=1g
Carbs=24g
Protein =4g

5.Beef Barley Vegetable Soup

Prep Time:20 mins

Cook Time: 4 hrs 15 mins
Total Time: 4 hrs 35 mins
Servings: 10

Ingredients

- 1 (3 pound) beef chuck roast
- ½ cup barley
- 1 bay leaf
- 2 tablespoons oil
- 3 carrots, chopped
- 3 stalks celery, chopped
- 1 onion, chopped
- 1 (16 ounce) package frozen mixed vegetables
- 4 cups water
- 1 (28 ounce) can chopped stewed tomatoes
- 4 cubes beef bouillon cube
- 1 tablespoon white sugar
- ¼ teaspoon ground black pepper, or more to taste

- salt to taste

Directions

1. Put the roast chuck in the slow cooker. Cook for 4 to 5 hours on High, or until tender. Cook for a another hour after adding the barley and bay leaf.

2. Remove the meat and cut it into small pieces. Throw away the bay leaf. Put the barley, meat, and broth aside.

3. Place a big stock pot over medium-high heat to preheat the oil. For five to seven minutes, sauté carrots, celery, onion, and frozen mixed vegetables until they are soft.

4. Add the beef-barley-broth combination, sugar, 1/4 teaspoon pepper, sugar, stewed tomatoes, and beef bouillon cubes. Boil for ten to twenty minutes, then lower the heat and simmer.

5. Before serving, season with salt and pepper.

Nutritional value

Calories=321
Fat=17g
Carbs=22
Protein =20g

6.Spring Vegetable Soup

Prep Time:15 mins
Cook Time:45 mins
Total Time: 1 hr
Servings:6

Ingredients

- 1 tablespoon vegetable oil
- ½ cup chopped onion
- 1 medium potato, peeled and chopped

- ½ cup chopped broccoli
- ½ cup frozen corn
- ½ cup torn spinach
- ½ cup chopped fresh mushrooms
- ½ cup chopped carrots
- ¼ cup chopped cabbage
- 2 (32 fluid ounce) containers chicken broth
- 6 ounces egg noodles
- 1 cup canned white beans

Directions

1. In a big pot, warm the oil over medium heat. Add the garlic and onion and sauté until softened. Add the potato, carrots, broccoli, corn, spinach, mushrooms, and cabbage and stir. Add the chicken broth and heat until it boils. Once the potato is cooked, reduce heat to low and simmer for 20 minutes.

2. Add the white beans and egg noodles to the saucepan and cook for another 7 minutes, or

until the beans are heated through and the noodles are soft.

Nutritional value

Calories=246
Fat=5g
Carbs=41g
Protein =10g

7.Yummy Spicy Black Bean Vegetable Soup

Prep Time:15 mins
Cook Time:35 mins
Total Time: 50 mins
Servings:8

Ingredients

- 1 tablespoon vegetable oil
- 1 onion, chopped
- 2 carrots, chopped
- 2 teaspoons chili powder
- 1 teaspoon ground cumin
- 4 cups vegetable stock
- 2 (15 ounce) cans black beans, rinsed and drained
- 1 (8.75 ounce) can whole kernel corn
- ¼ teaspoon ground black pepper
- 1 (14.5 ounce) can stewed tomatoes

Directions

1. Heat oil in a big saucepan over medium heat. Cook onion, garlic, and carrots for 5 minutes, stirring periodically, or until onion is softened. Add the cumin and chili powder; simmer for one minute while stirring. Bring the stock, maize, pepper, and one can of beans to a boil.

2. Meanwhile, purée the remaining can of beans and the tomatoes in a food processor or blender, then transfer to a pot. Once the carrots are soft, reduce heat, cover, and simmer for ten to fifteen minutes.

Nutritional value

Calories=165
Fat=3g
Carbs=27g
Protein =8g

8.Chicken, Rice, and Vegetable Soup

Prep Time:20 mins
Cook Time:35 mins
Total Time: 55 mins
Servings:4

Ingredients

- 5 cups water, or more as needed, divided
- 1 (14.5 ounce) can chicken broth
- 2 skinless, boneless chicken breast halves - cut into cubes
- 3 medium carrots, chopped
- 3 stalks celery, chopped
- 1 medium onion, chopped
- 2 cubes chicken bouillon
- ⅓ cup uncooked white rice
- salt and pepper to taste

Directions

1. In a large saucepan over high heat, combine 4 cups water and chicken broth; bring to a boil. Add the bouillon cubes, onion, celery, carrots, and chicken. After the vegetables are soft, reduce the heat to low, cover, and simmer for about 15 minutes.

2. Add the rice and boil for 15 minutes or until the rice is cooked, adding up to 1 cup of water if needed. Add pepper and salt for seasoning.

Nutritional value

Calories=105
Fat=1g
Carbs=22g
Protein =3g

9.Italian Vegetable Soup with Beans, Spinach & Pesto

Servings:10

Ingredients
- 1 ½ tablespoons olive oil
- 1 large onion, cut into small dice

- 3 medium carrots, peeled and sliced 1/4-inch thick
- 3 medium celery stalks, sliced 1/4-inch thick
- 1 medium bell pepper (red or yellow), stemmed, seeded and cut into medium dice
- 1 pound all-purpose potatoes, unpeeled and cut into medium dice
- 1 (16 ounce) can petite diced tomatoes
- 2 (15.5 ounce) cans cannellini or other white beans, undrained
- 6 cups low-sodium chicken broth in can or carton
- 7 ounces loosely packed baby spinach
- 1 cup frozen green peas
- Salt and ground black pepper
- Prepared pesto (found in grocer's refrigerated section)

Directions

1. In a soup kettle, heat the oil over a medium-high heat. Add the onions and sauté for about 5 minutes, or until soft. Bring the chicken broth, celery, carrots, potatoes, peppers, tomatoes, and beans to a boil. For about 15 minutes, or until the vegetables are just cooked, reduce heat to low and simmer. Stir in the peas and spinach and boil for an additional 3 to 4 minutes, or until the spinach wilts. Use salt and pepper to season to taste. Spoon soup into dishes; garnish each serving with a dollop of pesto.

2. Pack soup in individual leak-proof containers for lunch. Toss in some pesto and reheat the soup in the microwave.

Nutritional value

Calories=214
Fat=7g
Carbs=31g

Protein =12g

10.Fat-Free Vegetable Soup

Prep Time:25 mins
Cook Time:35 mins
Total Time: 1 hr
Servings:12

Ingredients

- 14 cups water
- 2 onions, chopped
- 2 large carrots, sliced
- 2 potatoes, peeled and cubed
- 2 green bell peppers, diced
- 1 (28 ounce) can whole peeled tomatoes with liquid, mashed
- 1 tablespoon chicken bouillon powder
- ¼ teaspoon ground black pepper
- 2 teaspoons curry powder (Optional)
- 3 cups finely shredded cabbage

- 2 stalks celery, chopped
- 1 ½ cups cauliflower florets
- 3 teaspoons dried dill weed

Directions

1. Measure out the water in a big cooking pot and add the potatoes, onions, carrots, green peppers, mashed tomatoes, black pepper, and curry powder. Boil until carrots are soft, about 20 minutes.

2. Cook for a further 10 to 15 minutes after adding the shredded cabbage, chopped celery, cauliflower florets, and dill weed. Add more water and bring the soup to a boil if it's too thick. To taste, adjust seasonings.

Nutritional value

Calories=68
Fat=0

Carbs=15g
Protein =3g

Chapter 5

Lunch Recipes Ideas

1.Honey Balsamic Vinaigrette

Prep Time:15 mins
Total Time:15 mins
Servings:12

Ingredients

- ½ cup balsamic vinegar
- 1 small onion, chopped
- 1 tablespoon soy sauce
- 3 tablespoons honey
- 1 tablespoon white sugar
- ½ teaspoon crushed red pepper flakes
- ⅔ cup extra-virgin olive oil

Directions

1. Fill a blender with the vinegar, red pepper flakes, onion, soy sauce, honey, sugar, and garlic. Add the olive oil gradually while puréeing on high. Puree for an additional two minutes, or until thick.

Nutritional value

Calories=145
Fat=13g
Carbs=8g
Protein =0g

2. Quinoa Tabbouleh

Prep Time:15 mins
Cook Time:15 mins

Total Time: 30 mins

Servings:4

Ingredients

- 2 cups water
- 1 cup quinoa
- 1 pinch salt
- ¼ cup olive oil
- ½ teaspoon sea salt
- ¼ cup lemon juice
- 3 tomatoes, diced
- 1 cucumber, diced
- 2 bunches green onions, diced
- 2 carrots, grated
- 1 cup chopped fresh parsley

Directions

1. Boil the water in a pot. Add a dash of salt and the quinoa. After 15 minutes of simmering, lower the heat to low and cover. When it cools to room temperature, use a fork to fluff it up.

2. In the meantime, mix the tomatoes, cucumber, green onions, carrots, parsley, lemon juice, olive oil, and sea salt in a big bowl. Add cooked quinoa and stir.

Nutritional value

Calories=354
Fat=17g
Carbs=46g
Protein =10g

3.Chicken Meatballs and Spaghetti.

Prep Time:20 mins
Cook Time:45 mins
Total Time: 1 hr 5 mins
Servings: 8

Ingredients

Sauce:

- 1 (16 ounce) can crushed tomatoes
- 1 (8 ounce) can diced tomatoes
- 3 (6 ounce) cans tomato paste
- 2 ¼ cups water
- 1 tablespoon dried basil
- salt and pepper, to taste

Meatballs

- 2 pounds ground chicken
- 1 cup dry bread crumbs
- ½ cup grated Parmesan cheese
- 2 eggs, lightly beaten
- 2 tablespoons Italian seasoning
- salt and pepper, to taste
- cooking spray
- 1 (16 ounce) package whole-wheat spaghetti

Directions

1. In a large saucepan over medium heat, stir together the diced tomatoes, crushed tomatoes, tomato paste, water, and basil. To taste, add salt and pepper. While making meatballs, bring to a boil, lower heat, and simmer for 15 minutes.

2. In a medium-sized bowl, combine the ground chicken, bread crumbs, Parmesan cheese, eggs, Italian seasoning, salt, and pepper. Form into 1-inch balls. Coat a big skillet with cooking spray and heat it over medium heat. The meatballs should be browned all over. Once the spaghetti sauce is simmering, add the meatballs and cook for about 30 minutes, or until the meatballs' internal temperature reaches at least 160 degrees Fahrenheit (72 degrees Celsius).

3. Add a small amount of salt to a large saucepan of water and heat it to a rolling boil on high. After the water reaches a boiling point, add the spaghetti and bring it back to a boil. Simmer for about 12 minutes, or until the pasta

is tender but still firm to the bite. Empty. Over the cooked pasta, serve the meatballs and sauce.

Nutritional value

Calories=491

Fat=8g

Carbs=66g

Protein =42g

4.Chicken Parmesan Pasta Casserole

Prep Time:20 mins

Cook Time:1 hr 30 mins

Additional Time: 5 mins

Total Time: 1 hr 55 mins

Servings:10

Ingredients

- 1 (16 ounce) package uncooked rotini pasta
- 1 pound skinless, boneless chicken breasts, cut into bite-size pieces
- 2 cups vegetable oil for frying
- 2 cups flour
- 4 large eggs, beaten
- 2 cups Italian seasoned bread crumbs
- 2 tablespoons garlic powder
- 1 (16 ounce) package shredded mozzarella cheese, divided
- 1 ½ (32 ounce) jars marinara sauce
- ½ cup dry red wine (such as Sangiovese)

Directions

1. Place a big saucepan of lightly salted water on high heat and bring it to a rolling boil. After bringing the water to a boil, add the pasta and stir again. Cook the pasta uncovered, tossing now and then, for about 8 minutes, or until it is cooked through but still firm to the biting. In a colander placed in the sink, thoroughly drain.

2.Preheat the oven to 350 degrees Fahrenheit (175 degrees Celsius) and heat the oil in a deep fryer or big saucepan to 375 degrees Fahrenheit (190 degrees Celsius).

3. Construct a breading area: Sort the flour, bread crumbs, and egg into three different bowls. Mix the bread crumbs with the garlic powder. Coat chicken in flour, dunk in egg, and then coat with bread crumbs while working in batches.

4. Gently cook the coated chicken in heated oil in small batches for 3 to 4 minutes, or until it turns golden brown and loses its pink center. When placed in the center, an instant-read thermometer should read at least 165 degrees Fahrenheit (74 degrees Celsius). Pat fry chicken dry with paper towels.

5. In a big bowl, mix cooked spaghetti, fried chicken, half of the mozzarella cheese, and half of the grated Parmesan cheese. Add marinara sauce and stir. Fill the empty marinara sauce jar with red wine; shake the jar, cover it, and then pour the contents into the pasta bowl. Mix

everything together. Line a sizable casserole dish with the spaghetti mixture, then cover with aluminum foil.

6. Bake for half an hour in a preheated oven. Take off the aluminum foil and top with the remaining 1/2 cup of Parmesan and mozzarella cheese. Put the oven back in and bake for another 30 minutes or so, or until the cheese has melted.

7. Take out of the oven and give it a five-minute rest before serving. Warm up the food.

Nutritional value

Calories=900
Fat=66g
Carbs=92g
Protein =30g

5.Broccoli Cheese Bake

Prep Time:15 mins
Cook Time: 30 mins
Total Time: 45 mins
Servings: 7

Ingredients

- 8 cups fresh broccoli
- ½ cup butter
- 2 tablespoons all-purpose flour
- 1 small onion, chopped
- 1 ¼ cups milk
- salt and pepper to taste
- 4 cups shredded Swiss cheese
- 2 large eggs, beaten.

Directions

1. Set the oven's temperature to 325°F, or 165°C.

2. Add broccoli to a steamer and cover it with one inch of boiling water. Simmer for two to six minutes, or until soft but not mushy. Empty.

3. In a medium saucepan over medium heat, melt butter. Stir in flour and fry until bubbling. Add onion and whisk in milk. After reaching a boil, cook for one minute. Take off the heat and add some salt and pepper.

4. Incorporate cheese and eggs, stirring until the cheese melts. Stir in broccoli until well mixed. Fill a 9 x 13-inch casserole dish with the ingredients.

5. Bake for about 30 minutes in the preheated oven, or until bubbling.

Nutritional value

Calories=441
Fat=33g

Carbs=15g

Protein =23g

6.Baked Salmon with Coconut Crust

Prep Time:10 mins

Cook Time:15 mins

Total Time: 24 mins

Servings:4

Ingredients

- 4 (4 ounce) salmon filets, skin removed
- 1 tablespoon lime or lemon juice
- ½ cup panko (Japanese bread crumbs, available in the Asian food aisle), or substitute dry bread crumbs
- ¼ cup flaked sweetened coconut
- Salt and freshly ground pepper, to taste
- Cooking spray

Directions

1. Set the oven's temperature to 425 F (220 C).
2. Arrange the salmon fillets onto a nonstick baking sheet and drizzle with olive oil.
3. Combine panko, coconut, salt, and pepper in a shallow dish. Place each salmon filet back in the baking pan after coating it with panko. Place any remaining crumbs over each filet of salmon. Apply a layer of cooking spray.
4. Bake for 12 to 15 minutes in the preheated oven. Place under the broiler until the crust is golden brown, if desired.

Nutritional value

Calories=264
Fat=14g
Carbs=12g
Protein =24g

7.Quinoa Chard Pilaf

Prep Time:20 mins
Cook Time:20 mins
Total Time: 40 mins
Servings:8

Ingredients

- 1 tablespoon olive oil
- 1 onion, diced
- 2 cups uncooked quinoa, rinsed
- 1 cup canned lentils, rinsed
- 8 ounces fresh mushrooms, chopped
- 1 quart vegetable broth
- 1 bunch Swiss chard, stems removed

Directions

1. In a big pot, warm the oil over medium heat. Add the garlic and onion, and sauté for 5

minutes, or until the onion becomes soft. Stir in the mushrooms, lentils, and quinoa. Add the broth in a pourable form. Cook for 20 minutes with a lid on.

2. Turn off the stove. Add the shredded chard to the stew and stir gently. Once the chard has wilted, cover and let it sit for five minutes.

Nutritional value

Calories=224
Fat=5g
Carbs=37g
Protein =10g

8.Guacamole Turkey Burger

Prep Time:10 mins
Cook Time:15 mins

Total Time: 25 mins
Servings:6

Ingredients

- 8 Ball Park Hamburger Buns
- 2 tablespoons extra virgin olive oil

Burgers:

- 8 ground turkey breast patties
- 1 teaspoon kosher salt
- 1 teaspoon ground black pepper
- 1 teaspoon ground cumin
- 1 teaspoon sweet paprika
- 1 tablespoon extra virgin olive oil

Guacamole:

- 4 ripe avocados
- ¼ cup finely chopped green onion
- ½ lemon, juiced
- ½ lime, juiced

- 1 teaspoon chili powder
- 2 tablespoons favorite Mexican salsa
- kosher salt to taste
- Trimmings: as desired, such as mayo, lettuce, tomato, onion and pickles

Directions

1. Cut avocados in half lengthwise to create guacamole. Take out and dispose of the pit. Using a spoon, remove the avocado flesh into a bowl.

2. Use a fork to mash in the liquids, salsa, chili powder, and salt until it becomes nice and chunky.

3. Place plastic wrap on top and leave aside. (If you wish to prepare the guacamole an hour or so in advance, cover the bowl and refrigerate it to keep it fresh. The avocado browns when air gets it, so be sure to place plastic wrap on top of the guacamole to prevent browning.)

4.Combine the paprika, cumin, salt, and pepper in a bowl and mix well.

5.Apply olive oil to both sides of each patty and then top with a mixture of seasonings.

6. Cook patties in a skillet or grill pan over medium-high heat, covered, for 5 to 6 minutes on each side, or until no pink is visible. Add the cheese during the last minute or so of cooking, if using.

7. Apply melted butter to both sides of each bun and reheat in a separate skillet over medium-high heat for approximately 15 seconds on each side, or until lightly toasted.

8.Stuff patties into bottom of each sandwich, then top with guacamole and additional preferred toppings. Present a small amount of salsa alongside.

Nutritional value

Calories=618
Fat=30g
Carbs=48g

Protein =47g

9.Cassava Flour Tortillas

Prep Time:15 mins
Cook Time:15 mins
Total Time: 30 mins
Servings:4

Ingredients

- ½ cup lukewarm water
- ¼ teaspoon salt
- 1 cup cassava flour
- 2 ½ tablespoons vegetable oil

Directions

1. Line a tortilla press with two parchment paper pieces. Put aside.
2. Add salt to a dish of warm water and whisk until it dissolves.

3. In a bowl, combine flour, oil, and salt water. Using your hands, knead until a smooth dough forms. Transfer the dough to a clean surface and gently work it into a compact, crumble-proof texture. Divide into four equal parts, then roll each into a ball.

4. Turn the heat up to medium-high on a griddle. In the tortilla press, press one ball of dough between two pieces of parchment paper. Apply pressure. Carefully remove the top piece of parchment paper from the press by opening it. Carefully flip the tortilla onto your palm and remove the second piece of paper. Reposition the paper onto the tortilla press. Cook the pressed tortilla on the heated griddle right away. Cook until bubbles appear, then turn and continue cooking until browned on the other side. The tortilla will shatter if you flip it before bubbles appear. Continue with the remaining dough balls.

5. Serve right away or reheat in the microwave for 30 seconds at 600W while covered with a cloth.

Nutritional value

Calories=221
Fat=9g
Carbs=35g
Protein =0

10.German Lentil Soup

Prep Time:10 mins
Cook Time:8 hrs
Total Time: 8 hrs 10 mins
Servings:8

Ingredients
- 1.2 cups dried brown lentils, rinsed and drained

- 3 cups chicken stock
- 1 bay leaf
- 1 cup chopped carrots
- 1 cup chopped celery
- 1 cup chopped onion
- 1 cup cooked, cubed ham
- 1 teaspoon Worcestershire sauce
- ¼ teaspoon freshly grated nutmeg
- 5 drops hot pepper sauce
- ¼ teaspoon caraway seed
- ½ teaspoon celery salt
- 1 tablespoon chopped fresh parsley
- ½ teaspoon ground black pepper

Directions

1. Fill a 5- to 6-quart slow cooker with lentils. Stir in the ham, carrots, celery, onion, and bay leaf. Add Worcestershire sauce, nutmeg, caraway seed, spicy pepper sauce, celery salt, parsley, and pepper 2.Cook on Low for eight to ten hours with a cover on. Take off the bay leaf before serving.

Tips

Stovetop method: Put the lentils, ham, spices, and chicken stock in a stock pot. After bringing to a boil, simmer for 30 minutes over medium heat. Cook the onion, celery, and carrots for 15 minutes or until they are soft. If more water is needed to maintain a soup-like consistency, add it.

Nutritional value

Calories=221
Fat=2g
Carbs=34g
Protein =16g

Chapter 6

Delectable Desserts without the Discomfort

1.Baked Apple Roses

Prep Time:25 mins
Cook Time:45 mins
Total Time: 1 hr 15 mins
Servings: 2

Ingredients

- 1 large red apple, cored and very thinly sliced
- ¼ cup white sugar
- 1 teaspoon ground cinnamon
- 1 sheet frozen puff pastry, thawed
- ¼ cup melted butter

* 1 large egg
* 2 teaspoons water
* 1 teaspoon confectioners' sugar (Optional)

Directions

1. Set the oven's temperature to 400°F, or 200°C. Place an oven rack in the center of the oven. Grease two 6- to 8-ounce ramekins, then sprinkle with powdered sugar.

2. Arrange the apple slices, slightly overlapping if needed, on a dish that is suitable to use in the microwave. Cook in the microwave on high for 45 seconds or until the slices start to soften. Place a kitchen towel and plastic wrap over the platter.

3.In a small bowl, combine sugar and cinnamon.

4.Roll the puff pastry sheet to a thickness of less than 1/8-inch. Using a pizza cutter, make two rectangles that measure 3 by 12. Keep the remaining parts for a different use.

5. Drizzle dough with melted butter and liberally dust with cinnamon sugar. Arrange the apple slices slightly overlapped along the long edge of the dough, extending about 1/4 inch past the edge. To create a long "folder" of dough with the rounded edges of the apple slices exposed, fold the bottom half of the dough over the slices.

6. In a small bowl, beat together the egg and water. Apply egg wash to the dough's outside. Add some cinnamon sugar on top.

7. Roll the dough into a rose-shaped pastry, beginning at one end. Using the end of the dough strip, seal the roll. Place the roses in the ramekins that have been ready. Add a little cinnamon sugar.

8. Bake for about 45 minutes on the middle shelf of a preheated oven, or until nicely browned. After removing the ramekins with tongs, let them cool for five to ten minutes on a baking sheet. Take out the apple roses from the ramekins, allow them to cool completely on a

wire rack, and then dust them with confectioners' sugar to serve.

Nutritional value

Calories=1050
Fat=71g
Carbs=90g
Protein =12g

2.Cinnamon Honey Butter

Prep Time:5 mins
Total Time:5 mins
Servings:16

Ingredients
- ½ cup butter, softened

- ½ cup confectioners' sugar
- ½ cup honey
- 1 teaspoon ground cinnamon

Directions

1. Combine butter, honey, confectioners' sugar, and cinnamon in a medium-sized bowl. Beat till fluffy and light.

Nutritional value

Calories=99
Fat=6g
Carbs=13g
Protein =0

3.Tasty Banana Oat Cookies

Prep Time:10 mins
Cook Time:15 mins
Total Time: 25 mins
Servings:12

Ingredients

- 2 bananas, mashed
- ¼ cup milk
- 1 large egg, beaten
- 1 teaspoon honey
- ½ teaspoon vanilla extract
- 1 cup rolled oats, or as needed
- 1 teaspoon ground cinnamon
- ½ teaspoon baking powder
- ⅛ teaspoon salt

Directions

1. Set the oven's temperature to 350°F, or 175°C. Use parchment paper to line a baking sheet.

2. In a bowl, combine mashed bananas, milk, egg, honey, and vanilla. Add the baking powder, cinnamon, oats, and salt and stir until thoroughly mixed. If the batter is too runny, add extra oats.

3. Spoon batter into mounds on the prepared baking sheet, spacing them a few inches apart.

4. Bake for about 15 minutes, or until the sides are golden and the tops appear dry.

Nutritional value

Calories=55
Fat=1g
Carbs=10g
Protein =2g

4.Almond Strawberry Chia Seed Pudding

Prep Time:10 mins
Additional Time: 4hrs
Total Time: 4 hrs 10 mins
Servings:4

Ingredients

- 2 cups almond milk
- 1 (16 ounce) package fresh strawberries, hulled
- ½ cup chia seeds
- ¼ cup honey
- 1 teaspoon vanilla extract

Directions

1. In a blender, puree the strawberries and almond milk until smooth; transfer to a bowl. Mix the vanilla extract, honey, and chia seeds into the pureed strawberries.

2. Place plastic wrap over the bowl and chill for approximately four hours, or until set.

Nutritional value

Calories=209
Fat=6g
Carbs=37g
Protein =4g

5.Chia Coconut Pudding with Coconut Milk

Prep Time:10 mins
Additional Time: 20 mins
Total Time: 30 mins
Servings:6

Ingredients

- 2 cups sweetened coconut milk
- 6 tablespoons unsweetened coconut milk
- 1 tablespoon agave nectar, or more to taste
- ½ teaspoon vanilla extract
- ¼ teaspoon ground cinnamon
- 1 pinch salt
- ½ cup chia seeds
- ½ cup diced fresh strawberries (Optional

Directions

1.In a dish, combine the sweetened and unsweetened coconut milks, agave nectar, salt, cinnamon, vanilla extract, and whisk to incorporate the chia seeds. Let the mixture soak for at least 20 minutes, or cover the bowl with plastic wrap and keep it in the refrigerator for the entire night.

2. Stir pudding and add strawberries on top.

Nutritional value

Calories=243
Fat=22g
Carbs=11g
Protein =4g

6.Coconut Banana Pancakes

Prep Time:15 mins
Cook Time:15 mins
Additional Total Time: 10 mins
Total Time:40 mins
Servings:15 mins

Ingredients

Pancakes:

- 1 ½ cups all-purpose flour

- 1 tablespoon white sugar
- 2 ¾ teaspoons baking powder
- 1 teaspoon salt
- 1 ¼ cups milk
- 1 egg
- 1 teaspoon vanilla extract
- 1 overripe banana, mashed
- 2 tablespoons butter, melted
- 1 teaspoon vegetable oil, or as needed

Syrups:
- 1 cup white sugar
- ¾ cup buttermilk
- 7 tablespoons butter
- 1 teaspoon coconut extract
- ½ teaspoon baking soda

Directions

1. In a bowl, combine flour, baking powder, salt, and 1 tablespoon white sugar. In a separate bowl, combine the egg, milk, and vanilla

essence. To incorporate the milk mixture, stir it into the flour mixture.

2. Using an electric mixer, beat banana in a bowl until it's smooth and creamy. Then, incorporate the banana cream into the batter. Blend the batter with melted butter. Batter should be chilled for ten minutes.

3. In a skillet over medium heat, heat the oil. Using big spoons, drop the batter into the hot oil and fry for 3 to 5 minutes, or until bubbles form and the edges are dry. In 3 to 5 minutes, flip, and continue cooking until the other side is browned. Proceed with the leftover batter.

4. In a saucepan over medium heat, combine 1 cup white sugar, buttermilk, and butter until sugar is dissolved. After one minute of boiling, lower the heat and stir in the baking soda and coconut essence. Simmer for one to two minutes, or until baking soda is dissolved.

Nutritional value

Calories=193
Fat=8g
Carbs=27g
Protein =3g

7.Fresh Yummy Strawberry Scones

Prep Time:30 mins
Cook Time:20 mins
Additional Time:25 mins
Total Time: 1 hr 15 mins
Servings:8

Ingredients

- 1.1 cup ripe strawberries - cleaned, hulled, and diced
- 1 teaspoon vanilla extract

- ½ cup light cream
- 2 cups all-purpose flour
- ⅓ cup white sugar
- 1 tablespoon baking powder
- ½ teaspoon salt
- ¼ teaspoon ground nutmeg
- 1 ½ teaspoons lemon zest
- 6 tablespoons cold unsalted butter, cut into chunks

Directions

1. Set the oven's temperature to 425 F (220 C). Use parchment paper to line a baking sheet.

2. To absorb fluids, arrange chopped strawberries on paper towels. In a small pitcher, combine cream and vanilla essence.

3. In a mixing basin, combine flour, sugar, baking powder, salt, nutmeg, and zest from the lemon. Using a pastry blender, cut in butter until the mixture is the consistency of coarse pea-sized crumbs. Add strawberries and mix lightly to combine.

4. Create a hole in the center of the mixture of flour. After swiftly stirring the dough until it's barely combined, pour the cream mixture into the hole. Give the dough two minutes to rest.

5. Work the dough for 4 to 5 minutes, or until it is satiny and smooth, on a lightly floured surface. Once the baking sheet is ready, transfer the dough there and pat it into an 8-inch round. Cut the circle into eight wedge-shaped pieces with a serrated knife. Arrange the wedges on the baking sheet, allowing a minimum of half an inch to separate them.

6. Bake for 16 to 18 minutes, or until the tops are lightly browned and crusty, in a preheated oven. Before serving, move to a wire rack and allow to cool for 20 minutes.

Nutritional value

Calories=232
Fat=9g

Carbs=34g

Protein =4g

8.Healthier Creamy Rice Pudding (EOE PRESCRIBED).

Prep Time:10 mins

Cook Time:1 hr 10 mins

Total Time: 1 hr 20 mins

Servings:4

Ingredients

- 1 ½ cups water
- ¾ cup uncooked brown rice
- 2 cups low-fat milk, divided
- ⅓ cup white sugar
- ¼ teaspoon salt
- 1 large egg, beaten
- ⅔ cup raisins

- 1 tablespoon butter
- ½ teaspoon vanilla extract

Directions

In a saucepan, combine the rice and water over high heat; bring to a boil. After 45 minutes or so, reduce heat to medium-low, cover, and simmer until soft.

2. In a clean saucepan, mix cooked rice, 1 1/2 cups milk, sugar, and salt. Simmer for 15 to 20 minutes over medium heat, or until thick and creamy.

3. Stir in raisins, beaten egg, and remaining 1/2 cup milk. Add 2 more minutes of cooking and stir regularly. Take off the heat and mix in the vanilla and butter. Warm up and serve.

Nutritional value

Calories=363
Fat=6g

Carbs=69g

Protein =9g

9.Poached Pears with Apricot Sauce

Prep Time:15 mins

Cook Time:25 mins

Total Time: 40 mins

Servings:12

Ingredients

- 1 ½ cups water
- ¾ cup white sugar
- ½ teaspoon vanilla extract
- 6 Bosc pears - peeled, halved and cored
- 1 cup apricot preserves
- 2 tablespoons cornstarch
- 2 tablespoons water
- ½ cup rum

Directions

1. In a saucepan over high heat, bring 1 1/2 cups water, sugar, and vanilla extract to a boil. After adding 3 or 4 pear halves, turn down the heat to medium, and simmer the pears gently for about 5 minutes, or until they have just turned soft. Cook the remaining pears in the same manner. Transfer the cooked pears to a warm chafing dish or metal serving dish.

2. Bring the syrup to a boil over medium-high heat, until it reduces to one cup. Return to a boil after stirring in the apricot preserves. Stir the cornstarch into the simmering syrup after dissolving it in two teaspoons of water. Cook for 30 seconds or until clear and thickened, stirring occasionally.

3. To serve, cover the pears with the hot sauce and top with the rum. Turn down the lights and carefully light the rum at the table. Serve when the alcohol has burned off.

Nutritional value

Calories=182
Fat=0g
Carbs=42g
Protein =0g

10.Rhonda Yummy Chocolate Pudding

Prep Time:10 mins
Additional Time:1 hr
Total Time: 1 hr 10 mins
Servings:4

Ingredients

- 1 avocado - peeled, pitted, and cut into chunks

- 1 banana, peeled and cut into chunks
- 1 cup unsweetened soy milk
- ¼ cup raw cocoa powder
- 2 tablespoons agave nectar
- 1 teaspoon lemon juice
- ¼ cup shredded unsweetened coconut (Optional)

Directions

1. In a blender, combine the avocado, banana, soy milk, cocoa powder, agave nectar, coconut, and lemon juice. Put a lid on and blend until smooth. Split into little jars and refrigerate for one hour to solidify.

Nutritional value

Calories=271
Fat=17g

Carbs=30g
Protein =4g

Conclusion

As we get to the close of our analysis of the senior-friendly Eosinophilic Esophagitis cookbook, it's important to assess all the information and useful recommendations we have learned. We've covered every aspect of dealing with end-of-life challenges as seniors in this extensive book, from comprehending the effects of stress to adopting mindful eating practices and everything in between.

This cookbook is based on a strong belief that seniors with end-of-life experience should be empowered to take control of their health and well-being. We've figured out trigger foods, negotiated the complexity of dietary limitations, and provided innovative fixes to make mealtimes meaningful and pleasurable. We have acknowledged the critical role that mental and emotional health play in the management of end-of-life concerns by highlighting the significance of stress management approaches.

Seniors can embark on a journey of resilience and self-discovery by taking up calming hobbies, asking friends and family for support, and developing mindful eating practices. The recipes, tips, and advice in this cookbook provide seniors dealing with end-of-life issues a glimmer of hope and inspiration.

Let's take the knowledge and wisdom this adventure has given us with us and apply it to our everyday lives as we wish it farewell. Let us welcome every meal as a chance to nurture our bodies and souls, and let us bravely and gracefully confront stress head-on. We pledge to succeed amid the Era of Encroachment and will always bolster one another.

I sincerely hope you use this recipe as a reliable guide to reach your highest level of health and vigor. Recall that you are not by yourself. We can get past EoE and fully appreciate life's blessings if we are persistent, determined, and a little creative. Cheers to good health, wonderful food, and the enduring resilience of the human spirit. My dear, I hope you enjoy reading! Greetings and enjoy your meal!